# ESSENTIAL OILS

# FOR

# BEGINNERS

THE COMPLETE GUIDE TO THE ESSENTIAL OIL FOR WEIGHT LOSS, BETTER SLEEP, DEPRESSION, DETOX, CLEANSE AND AROMATHERAPY

Renny Frost

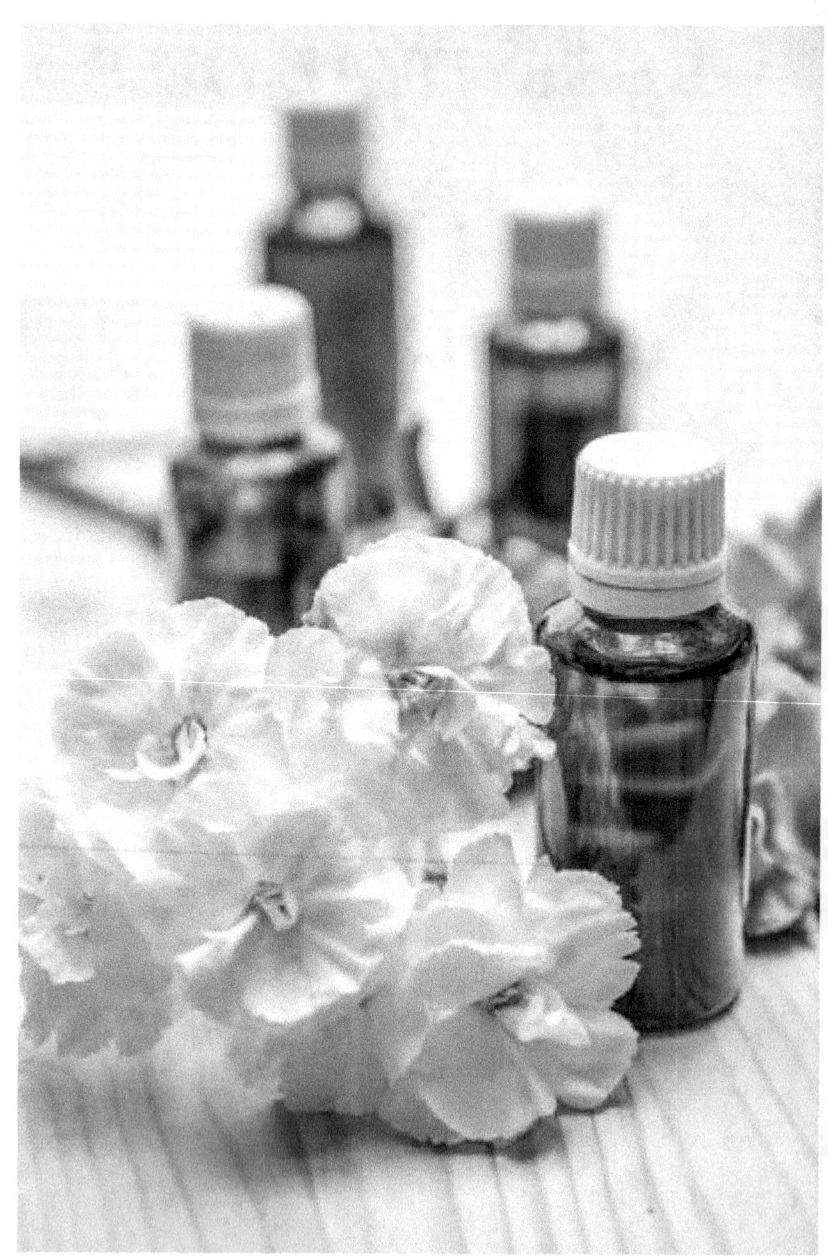

# INTRODUCTION

Recently, there has been increased interest in the possibilities of using essential oils. This interest has coincided with the belief that there have to be alternatives to the dominant medication approach, which has been used by healthcare professionals as the go-to solution for any ailments. Essential oils are perceived to be part of a wider campaign of health promotion and preventative measures that keep people away from hospitals. So what is an essential oil? Perhaps, the easiest way to define it is to consider how the core oils are made. The compounds that are used are, typically, derived from natural plants. Some literature refers to it as aetherolea, which is an extract from a given unit of flora. If you discover the term "ethereal oil", do not get confused, because it is merely a technical way of saying essential oil. The list of plants from which essential oils can be extracted is virtually endless. For example, you can get it from a clove of garlic or stem of thyme. The term "essence" is not just about the utility of the final product, but also the production process. In this case, you are capturing the essence or core element of a plant and then carrying it to the human body, using an intermediary element. The fragrance is very important, and the expectation is that it will broadly reflect what the plant smells like in its natural environment.

It is important to note that essential oils are not really indispensable. Therefore, it would be rather silly to compare them to something like an amino acid or even a fatty acid. The body cannot do without these, yet the essential oils are dispensable. Many people in the world have gone through life without ever using them. An organism has no important nutritional requirements that demand the inclusion of essential oils. Indeed, that is why some people see them as an indulgence for those who are looking for an alternative lifestyle. The most efficient way of extracting essential oils is through a process, known as distillation. The element that is the preferred choice for separating the various plant constituents is steam. The first stage is known as expression in which the plant or fruit begins to give off whiffs of the oils. These are linked to a carrier through solvent extraction. The high end point is the technically demanding absolute oil extraction. In the penultimate stage, there is a process of resin tapping, which also requires separate technical competencies. Finally, cold pressing allows us to get the essential oils in the forms in which they are readily available in the market today. There are a range of uses to which these extracts can be put to, the most obvious being fragrances. They also help in developing high end soaps, as well as a plethora of cosmetics. In dietary terms, essential oils have been used when flavoring drinks and other types of food. There are some households that use essential oils for the purpose of cleaning, as well as scenting areas in order to control bad odors.

Mainstream skin and body care products aren't for everyone. In fact, they are often full of so many processed ingredients that they cause more problems than they solve. If you have been interested in learning about how you can use essential oils to create your skin and body care products at home, or if you are looking for a larger variety of things that can be done with your essential oils, this book is going to provide the information you are looking for.

Starting with a brief lesson on what essentials are, how to use them and some precautions that you should know before investing in any essential oils, this book is going to go much deeper. This book is going to go in-depth on the best essential oils for many different beauty problems that people face, as well as the essential oils that cater to the many different skin types that people can have.

Aging is a natural part of life but one that often happens earlier in our life than we would like it to. Wrinkles, scars, stretch marks and varicose veins are all things that can be lightened and reversed with the use of essential oils, and this book is going to show you which essential oils are best for each of these applications.

We aren't going to stop there. We are also going to cover hair care, as well as some other applications for essential oils, including using them to relieve the effects of depression, anxiety and many frequent coughs, cold and sinus symptoms.

Did you know that everything you use around the house can affect your health? This book is also going to have a look at some of the products you are using around your house and how you can replace those products with homemade products using essential oils. The things you can do with essential oils are limitless, and this book is going to explore many of the options that are available to you!

This book is laid out in easy to read chapters that are loaded with the information you are looking for, when it comes to essential oils and numerous recipes that show all the ways they can be used. Thank you for purchasing this book, and it is my sincere hope that it will answer all your questions on essential oils.

# Table of Contents

# Chapter 1:
# WHAT ARE ESSENTIAL OILS?

Before we delve into what essential oils can do for you, we are going to take a quick minute to explain what exactly essential oils are, how they are made and how to choose your essential oils. This is going to help you later on when you are creating your recipes, and to make sure you have the foundation you need to understand fully how those recipes are going to work for you.

## What Are Essential Oils?

The term "essential oil" stems from the original term "quintessential oil." This dates back to the Aristotelian idea that all matter is composed of four elements: fire, water, earth, and air. Quintessence was considered to be a fifth element which was deemed to be the spirit or life force. Evaporation and Distillation were thought to be processes which removed the sense from the plant. This reflects in our modern day language where we use the term spirits to describe beverages such as whiskey and brandy.

An essential oil is an oil that occurs naturally in a plant or other source. It is typically obtained by distillation and has the characteristic fragrance of the plant it was extracted from.

## Expression

Also referred to as cold pressing, Expression is a method of extraction that is unique to citrus essential oils. Some of the oils that would use the phrase extraction method are a lemon, sweet orange, tangerine, bergamot, and lime. While expression used to be done by hand, we now use a more modern, and less labor intensive process today. During the process of expression, the rind of the fruit is placed into a container that has spikes that will puncture the fruit peel as the device is rotated. This technique is accomplished using centrifugal force. The spinning and puncturing release the essential oil that is then collected in a small area below the container. Spinning in a centrifugal force causes most of the essential oil to separate from the fruit juice.

## Choosing Essential Oils

Many people today, tend to be frugal and want to stretch their dollar as far as they can. However, this isn't always the best idea when it comes to essential oils. As you can see from the description on how essential oils are produced, it takes a lot of a plant to make a small amount of the oil. It stands to reason that essential oils, at least pure essential oils are going to be pricier.

In fact, to make one pound of the essential oil lavender, it takes one hundred pounds of the purple plant. On a more end, it takes four thousand pounds of Bulgarian roses to make just one pound of the essential oil.

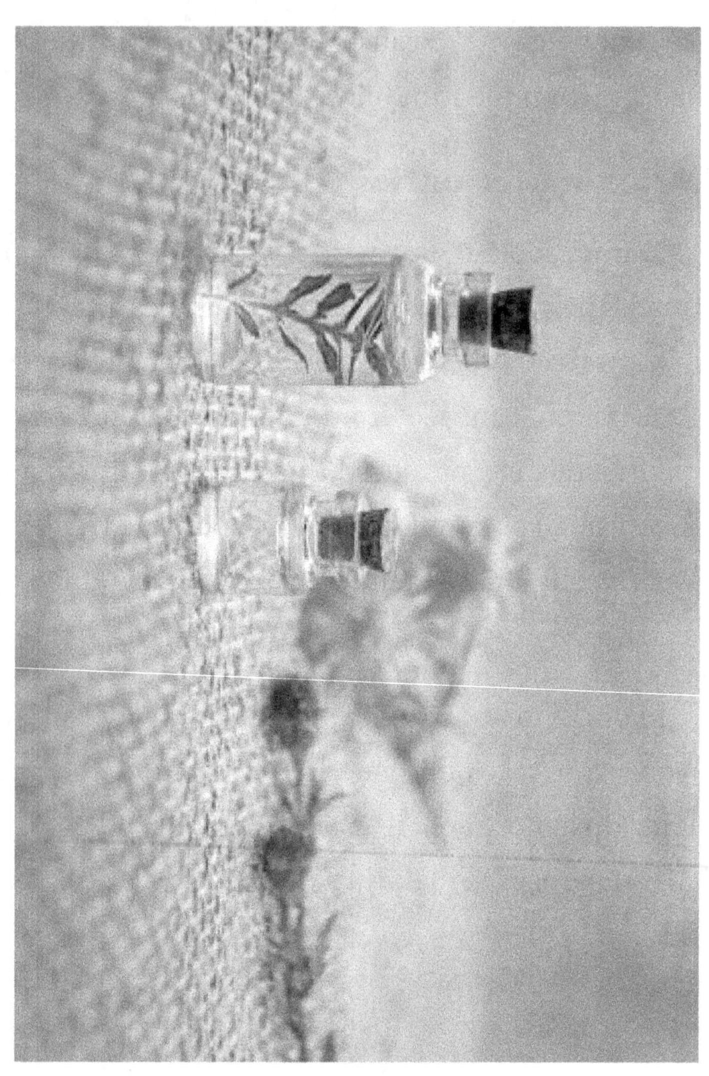

# Chapter 2:

# DIFFERENT ESSENTIAL OILS AND THEIR USES

## Carrier Oils

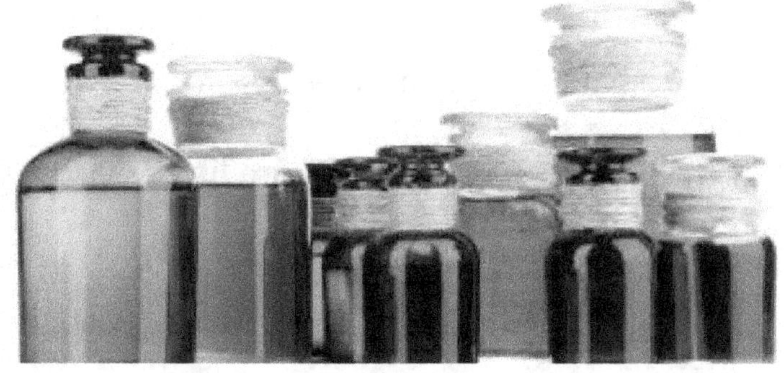

Carrier oils are the base oils that are used to dilute essential oils in recipes. In this chapter, we are going to look at the carrier oils that you can use with your essential oils as well as their properties. Most recipes will allow you to use your choice of carrier oil, so it is important to know what your options are, and what is going to work best for you and the recipe you are using. We are going to list consistency, absorbency, aroma, shelf life and any other pertinent characteristics you should know about each carrier oil.

It is important that you use a carrier oil to dilute your essential oils, as essential oils are very concentrated and can cause skin irritation if you don't. This is also true when you are using your essential oils in a distilled or to inhale. Continuously inhaling essential oils without diluting them first can lead to stripping the mucous membranes in your lungs.

As well as the carrier oils that are listed below, you can also use any lotion that you like as long as it is not made with petroleum-based oils or synthetic fragrances. The lotion is a good choice when you are looking for something with fast absorption. Because the lotion quickly absorbs, it is an excellent choice for injuries like sore muscles and joints.

## Lavender Flower:

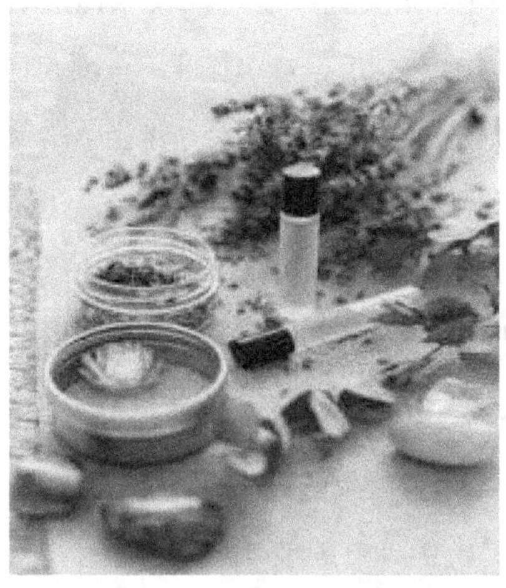

Perhaps, there is no plant more associated with sweet, elderly ladies than this one. However, you will be amazed at the range of uses to which the lavender essential oils can be put to. For example, it can be used to remove bad odors from bathrooms. It is also a core component of many high-end perfumes. Others have found ways of using it during their cooking, much to the surprise of those who cannot quite get around the idea that Lavender would taste good. The oils that have been extracted from it are potentially harmful. For example, they are known to be anti-androgenic in nature, as well as being estrogenic. These are very technical terms, for the impact that these oils have on pregnant women, as well as boys, who are still in their prepubescent stage of growth. Because they affect the hormonal balances of the body, it is not a good idea to start using lavender essential oils without consulting an expert, particularly, if you fall into the category that is most at risk. Nevertheless, there are new discoveries, concerning what lavender oils can do. For example, it has worked well for people, who want to get effective, but non-irritant insect repellent.

## Hazelnut Oil

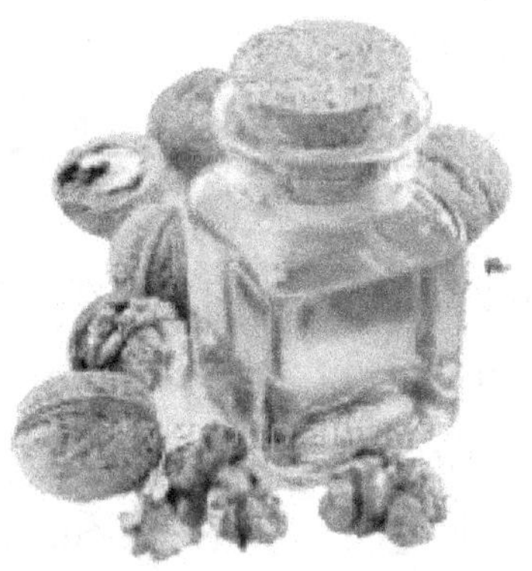

Consistency: Liquid.

Absorbency: Quickly absorbs and leaves a non-greasy feeling on skin.

Aroma: Very mild scent.

Shelf Life: Two years when refrigerated.

Best Uses: Massage and aromatherapy, skin care.

Other Facts: Deeply penetrating and stimulating to the circulatory system, and it also helps to tone and tighten the skin.

Hazelnut oil is created from both roasted as well as raw pressed hazelnuts. This oil is typically pale yellow in color. The natural fats in hazelnut oil are great for moisturizing and conditioning the skin, leaving it soft while decreasing the appearance of fine lines.

Hazelnut oil can be used in addition to sunscreen as it can assist in filtering the sun's rays. Hazelnut oil has a high content of catechins and tannins which make it an excellent choice for all skin types from the most sensitive and dry skin to the oiliest and acne ridden skin.

# Tea Tree Essential Oil:

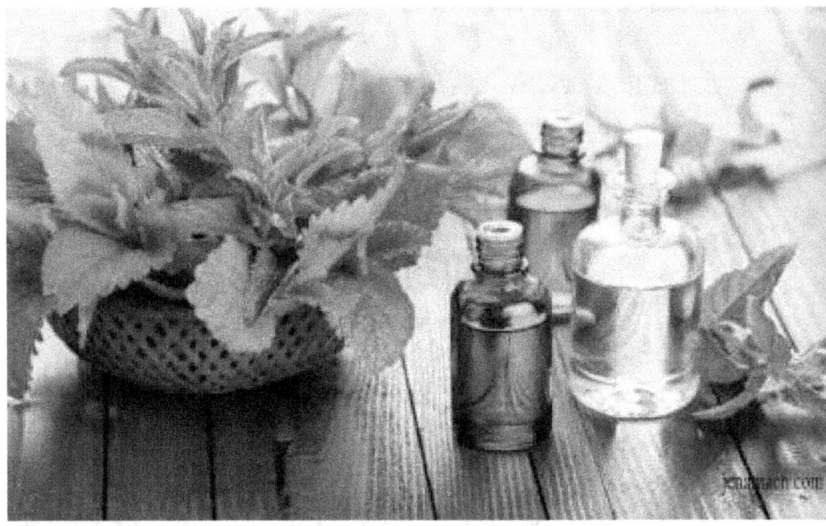

This essential oil is an antibacterial which helps to ward off the bacteria that cause acne. Tea tree essential oil also regulates oil production which contributes to decrease in the sensitivity of the skin and the number of breakouts that occur.

Botanical Name – Melaleuca alternifolia

Color – Clear with a yellow tinge

Perfumery Note – Middle

# Chapter 3:

# APPLICATION OF ESSENTIAL OILS

Essential oils can be used in four ways, these are:

1. *Aromatically*
2. *Topically*
3. *Internally*
4. *Externally*

## How to choose the application method:

The application method that is selected must meet the desired effect. Some essential oils make your skin irritated. Those essential oils need more dilution and can be used for the purpose of inhalation only.

## 1. STEAM

For the steam method, pour few drops of essential oil into steaming bowl which will quickly vaporize all the oil. Then, place a towel over the bowl of steam and your head and start breathing deeply. When using this method, it is advised to close your eyes as the method is very intense and direct.

The use of eucalyptus in the essential oil is helpful for the respiratory system and also helps with sinus problems. It is strongly recommended that this method should not be used by children under the age of 7 years.

Example, Cardamom used in steam evaporation methods.

## 2. SPRAY

Drops of essential oil can be mixed with water into a water-based solution. The mixture should be poured into a spray bottle and shaken for few minutes. Then, spray into the air. It is important to make sure that the mixture in the spray bottle has been mixed correctly for the required results.

# Application of essential oils topically

## To make the solution

Essential oil can only be used in diluted substance with only three to five percent concentration. This means that you take one teaspoon of the carrier, and add three drops of essential oils to it. This will make a solution of three percent.

When using essential oil for massage purposes, the application of it will be for a larger area, so only a one percent solution should be made. That means only one drop of essential oil should be added to a larger area of the body. For use with infants, only 0.25% solution should be added.

## Kind of carrier oil used in the solution

Carrier oils are available in the food stores or the stores where natural bath items are available. Organic and cold-pressed carrier oil are better to use, like apricot kernel oil, sweet almond oil, grape seed oil, jojoba oil or avocado oil. These oils contain the unyielding smell, and they should be refrigerated until they are used.

For wounds, the essential oil can be applied gently to the skin. These oils can be used in different ways. For example, for cuts and minor burns, real lavender essential oil can be utilized. Lavender can also be employed for the purpose of sleep and relaxation also.

It is one of those few essential oils that can be used on the skin directly without the process of dilution.

# Other techniques

## Compress

The essential oil can be used by doing a dilution process in which the oil is diluted with a liquid carrier, which can be water or oil and directly used in the affected area of skin.

For example, drops of ginger essential oil can be poured into the hot water and mixed well. Then a cloth can be soaked in that mixture, and used on the affected joint.

## Gargle

A few drops of essential oil can be poured into the water and mixed well. Rinse with the solution and spit it out. Repeat the process. This may help to heal a sore throat or other ailments.

## Bath

Use few drops of essential oil in bath water, and mix it so that the oil disperses completely. This combines the absorption and inhalation methods. One can also use full cream milk and other water soluble liquids to make the essential oil entirely dispersant in the water.

## Massage

A few drops of an essential oil may be added to any natural carrier oil and can be applied to the skin areas with gentle rubbing. The massage mixture can be made with only one percent concentration of essential oil.

## Internal applications of essential oil

For internal applications, one can use several methods, including oral ingestion or suppositories. It is recommended that ingestion of essential oils may only be taken under the supervision of a licensed doctor or health care provider.

# Chapter 4:
# SAFETY AND PRECAUTIONS

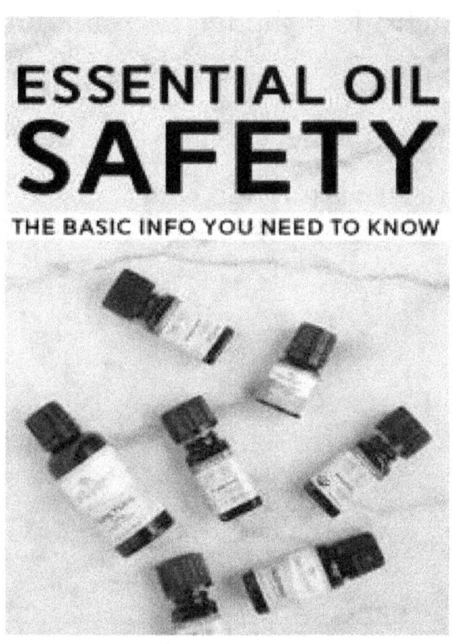


## Storage and Care

Essential oils are highly volatile plant oils, so, you must keep and store them properly so that they do not quickly lose their potency. However, real essential oils were distilled at temperatures of up to 140 degrees Fahrenheit, so leaving them out in a warm area will rarely alter their composition. They will return to their compressed state after cooling down. It is enough to store essential oils at room temperature.

Keeping them in a cooler will not result in prolonged shelf life or better preservation. If they do get cold and turn waxy or solid, do not force them to liquefy by applying heat. Allowing them to stand at room temperature is enough.

## Safe Use

Essential oils are dangerous to apply 'neat' or without a base. They are too concentrated and may irritate the skin. Also, it is easier to spread over vast areas if they are mixed with other oils that are safer to use on the skin and are also cheaper to use in large amounts. And because essential oils have volatile components, carrier oils contain these active ingredients so that they do not dissipate into the air, and are absorbed by the body. So, the chemical composition of the essential oil is retained.

Many essential oils that are sold in the market are already diluted in carrier substances. It is important to check the labels of products if they contain 100% of the oil or only a trace amount as this would affect any preparations.

## Ingestion and Contraindications

It is possible to overdose on essential oils taken internally. There is no evidence that ingesting of essentials oils orally is more efficient than inhalation or absorption through the skin. Though some oils are used in cooking and in preparations that may cause accidental swallowing (e.g., toothpaste, gargle), it is best to use them in small quantities and dilute in other edible and non-toxic substances.

Just because essential oils are natural, does not mean that they are not poisonous or harmful. They are highly concentrated, and anything in high doses will have an adverse effect. Synthetic oils are composed of human-made chemicals that are very toxic and should not be used in any food or oral preparations.

Nonetheless, pure essential oils are safe enough when used correctly.

## Adverse Reactions

A lot of people are allergic to even natural substances, and developing an allergic reaction to essential oils is possible. For example, a person with a known nut allergy (e.g., peanuts) should avoid all nut oils, especially because essential oils are concentrated versions of their plant sources. If unsure, it would be good to dilute an essential oil in a carrier oil and conduct a spot test on a small area of the skin. If no irritation develops in 24 hours, then the oil will be safe to use on the rest of the body.

# Chapter 5:
# ESSENTIAL OIL AND HEALTHY BENEFITS

## The oil and the beautiful

Ever since man began to be a part of social gatherings, his appearance became the most important thing for him. The skin, especially the facial skin turned out to be the first criteria for calling a man as "handsome" and a woman as "beautiful." In the modern era, the human race has started searching for beautifying and whitening miracles in synthetic chemicals which, in the long run, do more harm than good. Aromatherapy offers an entirely natural way of beautifying the skin and keeping it healthy with essential oils from plants. Listed below are different types of skin conditions, along with the oils that are most helpful.

## 1. Cracked/Chapped Skin

Cracked or Chapped skin results due to the lack of natural oils in your skin. Moreover, the soaps you use on your skin causes stripping of these natural oils from your bodies. One of the best essential oil to use for cracked and chapped skin is the Myrrh.

## 2. Dehydrated skin

You should use Lavender and Geranium to help you with dehydrated skin. These are great moisturizers for your dry and dehydrated skin, and you should use them in the winter months when not only the air outside is dry, but also when the heaters in your homes suck away all the moisture from your skin.

## 3. Eczema

The disease is often referred to as dermatitis. It is any itching or redness on your skin surface. Sometimes it gets alleviated through a change in the diet alone or simply by eliminating allergies. However, aromatherapy offers you two best oils for the treatment of eczema. These are Helichrysum and Thyme. The other useful essential oils include Lavender, Geranium, Tea Tree and Patchouli.

## 4. Impetigo

Impetigo is a skin condition in which "bumps" appear on your skin, which is filled with a yellowish liquid. It is a bacterial infection of the skin. Myrrh, Geranium, and Lavender are most useful essential oils for impetigo.

## 5. Scabies

Scabies appears as small, itchy bumps on the skin especially in the free skinned areas between the fingers and toes. In fact, these are little mites burrowing into different outer layers of your skin. Tea Tree and Peppermint have been found to be most effective against scabies.

## 6. Skin Ulcers

Skin ulcers or open sores of skin are not only ugly but also a potential home for infectious agents like bacteria. If you have a skin ulcer, you should protect it and thus, help it to heal. Myrrh and Lavender are best essential oils for skin ulcers.

## 7. Sunburn

All types of skin burns are soothed by Lavender in an efficient and natural way. Tea tree and Roman Chamomile can also help.

## 8. Callouses

Do you have a thick and flat skin, maybe on both of your feet? The essential oil that you can apply on it is Oregano.

## 9. Corns

These are mostly the result of wearing shoes that are ill-fitting. Clove is the best natural way of treating corns. However, you can also use Grapefruit and Peppermint for the same.

## 10. Diaper Rash

Do you have small kid's diapers rash? If yes, then you would surely want to keep Lavender essential oil around. The other essential oil found to be effective against diaper rash is Chamomile.

## 11. Fungal Infections

You might have heard about the Athlete's Foot. It is not some harsh sporty term, but merely a fungal infection on the skin, especially the toes. For almost all types of fungal infections of your skin, you should use Oregano and Tea Tree oils.

## 12. Itching/Rashes

Ever wondered what causes your skin to be extremely itchy?  It could be as a result of any allergy, dryness, the reaction of the skin to a laundry detergent or some other chemical you used in the kitchen or at work. For generalized itchiness, Lavender and Peppermint are best suited. For skin rashes, you can use Lavender and Tea Tree oils.

## 13. Scarring

For scar prevention, the aromatherapists recommend Rose and Frankincense. When scarring occurs after a burn or an injury, the best suited essential oil is the Lavender. Helichrysum has also been found to reduce the scars effectively. Other essential oils for the same purpose are Myrrh and Geranium.

## 14. Stretch Marks

Almost everyone gets stretch marks on their skin. You may be a pregnant woman who got them on your abdominal skin. You may be a previously large male who has reduced weight considerably so much that the stretch marks remain on different body parts. These are not harmful, but sometimes your skin stretches to the point of being sufficiently damaged. The two essential oils Myrrh and Lavender are best for reducing the stretch marks, and they also help your skin to heal.

## 15. Wrinkles

With your every birthday, nature gifts you a small line on skin. But the same nature has blessed you with the power of some useful oils for those wrinkles.

# BEST ESSENTIAL OILS FOR ANTI-AGING:

Essential oils are an excellent choice when you are looking for an anti-aging treatment that is going to work really, it isn't going to cost a lot of money and smells amazing. When you are purchasing over the counter anti-aging treatments, you are going to spend a lot more money, and these treatments often have ingredients in them that are unfamiliar.

When you are using essential oils on your face, and especially around your eyes, you need to be aware that the essential oil might react with the skin. Essential oils are a natural and healthy approach to countering the aging of our skin. In addition to all of the anti-aging benefits, these oils are also going to keep your skin smelling good throughout the day.

Many things can lead to premature aging of our skin. Smoking, alcohol use, sun exposure and a poor diet all contribute to wrinkles, age spots, and tired and dull looking skin. Here, we are going to cover some of the best essential oils for aging skin. Once we are familiar with the options of essential oils, we are going to look at some recipes that they can be used in.

## Lavender Essential Oil:

This essential oil contains anti-inflammatory, anti-aging, antifungal and antimicrobial properties. Lavender essential oil is ideal for delaying fine line wrinkles, age spots, and sun spots thanks to its regenerative properties.

Botanical Name – Lavandula augustifolia or Lavandula officinalis

Color – Clear with a tinge of yellow

Perfumery Note – Top to middle

# BENEFITS OF INHALING ESSENTIAL OILS

When essential oils are inhaled into the lungs, it brings both physical and psychological benefits. Here is a brief list of the advantages that can be found by inhaling essential oils along with the essential oils that can be used for each purpose.

## 1. Stress Relief:

- Lavender essential oil

- Frankincense essential oil

- Rose essential oil

- Roman Chamomile essential oil

- Vanilla essential oil

## 2. Sinus Congestion Relief:

- Tea Tree essential oil

- Eucalyptus essential oil

- Lavender essential oil

- Peppermint essential oil

- Oregano essential oil

## 3. Sore Throat Relief:

- Eucalyptus essential oil

- Rosemary essential oil

- Camphor essential oil

- Thyme essential oil

- Sage essential oil

## 4. Cough Relief:

- Tea tree essential oil

- Myrrh essential oil

- Peppermint essential oil

- Lavender essential oil

- Lemon essential oil

## 5. Bronchitis Relief:

- Lavender essential oil

- Frankincense essential oil

- Eucalyptus essential oil

- Peppermint essential oil

## 6. Anxiety Relief:

- Bergamot essential oil
- Frankincense essential oil
- Basil essential oil
- Sage essential oil
- Lavender essential oil
- Marjoram essential oil
- Ylang-ylang essential oil

## 7. Depression Relief:

- Lavender essential oil
- Rose essential oil
- Geranium essential oil
- Bergamot essential oil
- Sandalwood essential oil
- Marjoram essential oil
- Jasmine essential oil

## 8. Insomnia Relief:

- Lavender essential oil

- Marjoram essential oil

- Neroli essential oil

- Roman Chamomile essential oil

- Ylang-ylang essential oil

# Chapter 6:
# WHAT IS AROMATHERAPY?

Aromatherapy is an alternative medicine that uses essential oils to improve a person's health or mood. While many people consider this type of treatment to be irrational and wishful thinking, there have been some scientific studies showing that aromatherapy is effective at making you feel good, although there was no evidence that it makes you well.

The essential oils that are used in aromatherapy have a different composition than other herbal products you can purchase. This is because the distillation that happens in aromatherapy recovers the lighter phytol molecules.

## How Does Aromatherapy Work?

It is commonly believed that the inhalation of essential oils stimulates the olfactory system, which is the part of the brain that is connected to smell. When this happens, a signal is sent to the limbic regime of the brain that is responsible for controlling emotions and retrieving learned memories which lead to memories to be released which will make a person feel relaxed, happy, calm, or even stimulated.

When we target our sense of smell with the essential oils, we are being affected emotionally. When we apply essential oils topically, we are activating thermal receptors and destroying microbes and fungi.

When you are using your essential oils topically, you are still taking advantage of the aromatherapy benefits that come with essential oils.

## Aromatherapy Blends

In the last chapter, we covered the different essential oils that can be used when you choose to inhale the essential oils. However, you aren't limited to using only one essential oil in these methods. You can also create blends that you can place on your pillow, in a diffuser, or in any of the other methods. For each of the blends, combine in a dark colored glass bottle. For these blends, you do not need carrier oil unless you are applying them to the skin.

## Insomnia Aromatherapy Blend:

- Ten (10) drops of roman chamomile essential oil.

- Five (5) drops of sage essential oil.

- Five (5) drops of bergamot essential oil.

## Anxiety Aromatherapy Blend:

- Ten (10) drops of bergamot essential oil.

- Ten (10) drops of sage essential oil.

- Five (5) drops of frankincense essential oil.

## Stress Relieving Aromatherapy Blend:

- Ten (10) drops of roman chamomile essential oil.

- Five (5) drops of lavender essential oil.

## Depression Aromatherapy Blend:

- Ten (10) drops of grapefruit essential oil.

- Five (5) drops of ylang-ylang essential oil.

- Five (5) drops of lavender essential oil.

## Congestion Aromatherapy Blend:

- Thirty (30) drops of eucalyptus essential oil.

- Twenty-Six (26) drops of myrrh essential oil.

- Four (4) drops of peppermint essential oil.

# Chapter 7:
# ESSENTIAL OILS FOR WEIGHT LOSS

## Fennel Oil

Fennel oil is earthy and sweet, and another essential oil that can help deal with weight loss and digestion problems. Besides improving the digestion and suppressing appetite, fennel essential oil provides more restful sleep. Fennel is a source of melatonin, so it helps you get your sleeping cycle right. helps you have the best sleep of your life every single night.

## How to Use Fennel Oil?

Inhale fennel essential oil diluted or make a mixture of 80 drops of fennel, 40 drops of bergamot, and 24 drops of patchouli oil and massage it on the abdomen for appetite suppression.

In your produce isle, fennel is that plant that looks a little like celery stalks with a feathery top that sounds like the trees from the children's book, and related movies, The Lorax. Fennel stalks are also tasty to eat raw or cooked, and they are highly nutritious. They are used in many Mediterranean cuisines, which are known to be some of the healthiest in the world. Fennel has a subtle sweet licorice taste. But I only recommend that you eat fennel in the season, because, it has a bitter and rotten taste and if you try it or tried it out of season, you may think you don't like it. That is why essential oils are so high. You can get the benefits all year round; because when essential oils are created, the benefits are preserved for months or even years to come.

## Lavender Oil

Lavender is another of the oils in use for thousands of years. It is used for culinary purposes as well as for health and beauty purposes. Lavender is often found in perfumes because it gives an adamant base for other scents. Lavender comes from the word "Lavare" (Italian), and it means, "to wash." This plant got its name thanks to the amazing aroma of the flowers, which smell, clean, fresh and vibrant.

Lavender is best known for its calming effects. It has a strong relaxing scent that helps us release any stress in no time. It's widely used for treating depression, migraines, headaches, emotional stress, etc. Scientists have thoroughly researched this great plant, so, the results are highly supported by substantial scientific data: lavender has an enormous impact on the autonomic nervous system and because of this asset; Lavender is used to treating insomnia and to stabilize heart rate. Researchers also show it even boosts cognitive functions, it fights anxiety, and it is very efficient in decreasing mental stress.

Weight gain has a lot to do with stress and sleep, as we have mentioned above, so lavender oil can help you to cope with stress and release built up tension in your body. Modern studies have shown that color shows better results when fighting insomnia than medicines again and again and again. People keep re-doing the studies. It is like some just can't believe how well it works and that it is  much better than leading prescription sleep aids, which often force your body into sleep mode leaving you feeling groggy the next day. If you ever watched the Wizard of Oz with Judy Garland, you remember the poppy field where everyone wanted to fall asleep.

Lavender is used in helping to treat irritation and inflammation throughout the body. When you are trying to lose weight, any inflammation in your body will prevent weight loss because our body is distracted by these "emergencies." Our bodies can be like team supervisors sometimes. If you have ever been a team lead, supervisor or manager, you will get this reference. They are rushing around, trying to put out fires to the point that they cannot get any work done. These fires in business are usually caused by inadequate oversight, planning and prioritizing. It is the same thing with our bodies. Poor planning and choices on our part lead to fires (inflammation), and when or agencies are busy with fires all day long, they cannot work efficiently to burn fat and give us the energy we need to get things done. Using the lavender essential oil can help you first, by improving your health, and then you can focus more on losing pounds.

Another benefit of using lavender essential oil is solving respiratory problems. Any throat infections, problems with breathing, coughing, asthma, can make losing weight harder because you are not breathing properly and there is not enough oxygen in your blood to supply the cells. Breathing is crucial because our body needs oxygen to function at its best, and if we breathe shallow, it is like driving a car with half-deflated tires. You are wasting a lot of gas, and you are wearing your tires out at the same time. Lavender essential oil can help you with respiratory problems, and it can improve your breathing capacity.

Lavender helps with the mobility of food in the intestine, and it promotes the production of gastric juices and bile, helping your indigestion and stomach/intestine problems such as gas, diarrhea, flatulence and vomiting. As we have already discussed, when our digestive system is working, as it should, we can absorb nutrients and lose weight.

## How to Use Lavender Oil?

If you have respiratory problems, inhale the vapor of lavender essential oil or rub a few drops on your abdomen. For insomnia problems put a few drops on your pillow, or leave a diffuser with lavender oil in your bedroom. If you have problems with digestion, add a few drops to a glass of water and drink it daily.

## Aromatherapy for Cellulite:

The usual causes of cellulite are consumption of chocolates, fast foods, caffeine, alcohol and smoking cigarettes as well as toxin build-up and a lack of exercise. The other causes which have been associated with this condition are fluid retention, poor circulation, hormones such as progesterone and estrogen, heredity, and aging. It has been seen that the cellulite usually develops during times of hormonal change in life like puberty, premenstrual, pregnancy and menopause. Recently, the researchers mainly say that the roots of cellulite development are in gender and genetics. Womenfolk have weaker collagen, a constituent of skin layers, than men. When the fat is stored in many tiny pockets surrounded by collagen, it tends to buckle under their weight. Thus, the fat cells start to pucker. This results in the formation of cellulite.

## How does aromatherapy help against cellulite?

Since poor circulation is strongly considered as a causative factor, thus, an excellent remedy for cellulite is the regular massaging with essential oils. This powerful method not only increases the circulation and leads to the elimination of toxins by helping you overcome lymphatic congestion in the area, but also helps in breaking up the ugly fatty deposits too, when massaging is done correctly. It also brings some cosmetic relief by toning and firming the skin and leaving it silky, smooth and beautiful.

## Oils that bust Cellulite

You can use the citrus oils like lemon as well as grapefruit for effective stimulation of your lymphatic system. You can also blend them with juniper berry for excellent results. Geranium oil has a balancing effect on your hormones. Other useful anti-cellulite essential oils are cypress, carrot seed, ginger, thyme white, rosemary, and lime.

# Chapter8:
# ESSENTIAL OILS FOR DEPRESSION

## The 50 Best Essential Oils for Stress Relief and Anxiety

The following are the top 50 essential oils that are known to provide therapeutic benefits for anxiety and stress. While there are virtually hundreds of other essential oils out there that can provide similar effects, the ones featured in this book are considered as the more traditional, and widely used varieties.

Note that the specific benefits vary from one essential oil to another, and it is therefore up to you to select the right essential oils to use base on your particular situation and preferences.

## 1. Amyris

The Amyris essential oil helps to promote inner strength and provides centering and balance when used with a diffuser. Although, popularly referred to as the West Indian Sandalwood, Amyris is not related at all to the real Indian sandalwood. The misconception probably stems from the fact that the plant from which the Amyris essential oil is extracted, has a slightly sweet, woody, and balsamic aroma that is similar to sandalwood.

Amyris is typically used to act as a fragrance fixative because it slows down the process of evaporation and dissipation of whatever scent it is blended with. It can be combined with other essential oils such as jasmine, cedarwood and rose to achieve maximum stress-relieving benefits.

## 2. Angelica

The name Angelica is derived from the word angel. According to folklore, the plant's various healing qualities were revealed to a monk at a time when there was a terrible plague ravaging the people.

Lab tests were conducted to compare the effects of the essential oil extracted from Angelica against diazepam, an anti-anxiety drug. Based on the results, the conclusion was that both angelica essential oil and diazepam provide anti-anxiety effects. It is important to note that, while both are effective treatments for anxiety, angelica – being natural and plant-based – is free from any unwanted side effects. And that should tilt the balance for the essential oil.

## 3. Anise

When used in a diffuser, anise produces a mildly euphoric and cheering effect; thus, helping relieve anxiety and stress. The essential oil extracted from anise and star anise are usually sold and used interchangeably. This is because the two produce the same aroma and have similar chemical makeups. Both have anethole as the primary constituent. Anethole is a sweet substance that turns solid at room temperature. When this happens, just warm the bottle up using warm bath water until the essential oil begins to liquefy.

## 4. Bay Laurel or Bay Leaf

Bay leaf essential oil is known to help provide mental balance, reduce nervous exhaustion, ward off feelings of anxiety and melancholy, induce peace and harmony, and boost self-esteem and confidence.

To use, just dilute 15 to 20 drops of bay laurel essential oil in your bath water, or 100 ml of your preferred base oil, or use it with a diffuser. The oil blends well with lemon, lime, orange, cypress, clary sage, juniper, hyssop, olibanum, labdanum rosemary, pine, and spice oils. While bay laurel may be used on its own, combining it with other essential oils will help increase the therapeutic benefits.

## 5. Basil

The essential oil extracted from basil is stimulating and refreshing. The Scientific name is Ocimum basilicum. It is typically recommended for mental exhaustion relief. Basil helps combat depression, anxiety, mental fatigue, irritability, and migraines, and likewise, provides a peaceful emotional state.

The following blend is recommended for optimum revitalizing and stimulating results: 7 drops of basil + 7 drops of bergamot + 3 drops of peppermint + 2 drops of lavender + 1 drop of eucalyptus.

# 6. Bergamot

Bergamot essential oil is known for its calming effects. Bearing the scientific name Citrus bergamia, it is also considered as a mood enhancer, equalizer, and modifier. The oil can be topically applied as a deodorant or added to water and food as a dietary supplement. Bergamot has a scent that is best described as sweet, citrusy, fruity, and lively.

Bergamot essential oil, however, can be sensitive to direct sunlight; thus, as a safety measure, if you intend to go outdoors in the next 24 hours, you should not apply it topically on your skin.

To achieve optimum benefits, bergamot can be blended with other essential oils such as cypress, chamomile, geranium, eucalyptus, juniper, jasmine, lemon, lavender, palmarosa, ylang-ylang, and patchouli.

# 7. Cardamom Seed

The essential oil extracted from cardamom seed produces a camphor-like and spicy aroma with some floral hints. Cardamom seed lends a warm note to floral perfumes and masculine scents. When inhaled, the essential oil provides a comforting, alluring and warming effect that results to reduced anxiety and stress levels.

Cardamom seed essential oil blends well with frankincense, bergamot, cedarwood, coriander, and ylang-ylang to provide optimum benefits for tension and anxiety.

## 8. Carrot Seed

Extracted and distilled from the seeds of conventional carrots, carrot seed essential oil replenishes, nourishes, and restores the spirit when inhaled using a diffuser. It can provide a soothing relief during highly stressful situations. It has a dry woody, earthy and somewhat sweet scent.

Carrot seed oil is usually used as an ingredient in various types of perfume such as fantasy, nature, and Oriental fragrance types because of the essential oil's single fatty-woody note. It is likewise a great oil to include in your stock of skin care oils.

# 9. Cedar wood

The scientific name for Cedarwood is Cedrus atlantica. The essential oil is noted for its calming qualities. It is known as a mood equalizer and enhancer with its soft, warm, and woody aroma. Clinical tests have proven that cedar wood offers significant benefits for children who have ADHD and ADD. It is interesting to note that cedar wood was used by Native Americans to communicate with spiritual beings.

Cedar wood essential oil stimulates the brain's limbic region (which is the center of emotions), as well as the pineal gland (which is responsible for the release of melatonin, an important player in establishing proper sleep cycles.) The oil can be topically applied or used with an essential oil diffuser. It combines well with other essential oils such as clary sage, bergamot, eucalyptus, cypress, juniper, floral oils, myrrh, rosemary, and frankincense. Cedar wood must be used with extreme caution by pregnant women to avoid complications.

## 10. Chamomile, German

Chamomile, specifically the German variety (scientific name Matricaria recutita) can help explain the mind, diffuse anger, and stabilize one's emotions. It can be inhaled or diffused. Like all essential oils with frequency around the 105 MHz levels, chamomile works well for the emotional aspect of the user. Its blend classification is personified. German chamomile has a rich, dark, herbaceous, and cocoa-like aroma.

The essential oil, however, can cause irritation on sensitive skin and must be used with caution by pregnant and lactating women. Chamomile is best combined with geranium, fir, hyssop, helichrysum, lemongrass, lavender, sandalwood, marjoram, spruce, tea tree, spearmint, and wintergreen.

## 11. Chamomile Roman

The scientific name of Roman chamomile is Chamaemelum Nobile. Tea made from the plant is known for its sleep-inducing properties. Just imagine how much more potent would  produce the essential oil, which is a lot more concentrated, when extracted from Roman Chamomile be. Roman chamomile essential oil provides wonderful relaxing and calming effects. It also helps reduce anger, lower anxiety levels, and release pent up emotions.

The essential oil can be diffused or applied at the back of the neck and on the temples (about two drops) when faced with stressful situations or just before bedtime. Roman chamomile is also recommended for meditation purposes and to help an individual express his true feelings (which can be achieved with topical application on the throat area.) The oil is classified as a personified blend and combines well with clary sage, geranium, rose, and lavender. It has an apple-like, sweet, fresh, and fruity-herbaceous aroma. Some words of caution, though. It may be irritating to sensitive skin, so it is recommended to dilute it with an equal part of vegetable oil such as almond and coconut oil before using.

## 12. Cinnamon

Cinnamon essential oil may be extracted from the tree's bark or leaves. When used in aromatherapy, it provides warming and soothing effects. Cinnamon bark oil or Ceylon cinnamon is the most commonly traded variety. It has an aroma similar to Chinese cinnamon or cassia, but Ceylon cinnamon is more preferred for use in perfumes because of its warm and floral-enhancing qualities. It is typically blended with frankincense and other essential oils with oriental woody notes.

On the other hand, cinnamon essential oil distilled from cinnamon tree's leaves has a scent that is more like that of cloves rather than the regular cinnamon. This is because the leaf extract contains a large volume of eugenol. Cinnamon leaf essential oil is usually used as an ingredient in Oriental perfumes. The oil, however, must be utilized with proper care since it is known to irritate the skin. In aromatherapy, cinnamon leaf oil helps revitalize and refresh.

## 13. Citronella

Citronella essential oil comes in two types: Java and Ceylon. While the grass from which the Java oil is extracted is cultivated in various parts of the tropics, the Ceylon variety is primarily grown in Sri Lanka, the former Ceylon. There are subtle differences between the essential oils extracted from the two grass types regarding aroma and composition.

The aroma of Ceylon citronella is somewhat grassy, warm-woody, and fresh. It is ideal for use in outdoor spray scents, room sprays, and various household products. On the other hand, the essential oil extracted from Java grass emits a more floral and sweeter aroma that is more appropriate for perfumery. Both citronella essential oils are known for their purifying and vitalizing properties.

## 14. Clary Sage

Clary sage was also the subject of various other studies, and most results indicated that indeed, the essential oil is beneficial in helping with anxiety.

While it cannot be clearly concluded that it is an effective cure, there are positive indications that the clary sage provides a soothing effect on the body and mind, although only on a temporary basis. And while more studies are needed to confirm this claim, many specialists say that the essential oil contains antidepressant properties as well.

## 15. Clove Bud

The best type of clove essential oil, is that which is distilled from the clove tree's whole dried flower buds. It has powerful comforting and warming properties when inhaled or used with an essential oil diffuser. While clove oil can also be derived from the stems and leaves of clove trees, the extracts are less potent.

Clove bud essential oil boasts of a strong, warm, spicy-fruity, and sweet smell. It should, however, be handled with extreme care as it can highly irritate the skin, specifically the more sensitive types.

## 16. Coriander

Coriander essential oil carries the scientific name Coriandrum sativum. It is popular for its uplifting properties. Coriander also helps fight anxiety, mental fatigue, excessive worrying, nervous tension, and depression.

The essential oil from coriander can be combined with cinnamon, bergamot, grapefruit, ginger, neroli, lemon and orange essential oils to achieve maximum uplifting and anxiety-reducing effects.

## 17. Eucalyptus

Eucalyptus essential oil helps promote the proper functioning of the nervous system. It fights stress, depression, anxiety, headaches, and extreme fatigue. It is known for its energizing and calming qualities.

Eucalyptus oil combines well with chamomile, cedarwood, cypress, ginger, geranium, juniper, grapefruit, lemon, lavender, peppermint, marjoram, rosemary, thyme, and pine essential oils.

## 18. Fennel, Sweet

The essential oil from sweet fennel exudes an earthy, anise-like, and very pleasant scent. This is attributed to the oil's main constituent – anethole. The substance is more abundant in fresh fennel than in bitter fennel oil.

When used with an essential oil diffuser and inhaled, sweet fennel essential oil provides restorative, nurturing, and supportive effects that that can help provide almost instant anxiety and stress relief.

## 19. Frankincense

Also known as Boswellia Sacra or Boswellia carterii, frankincense is a type of equalizer and enhancer essential oil that is a rich source of sesquiterpenes, molecules that have the ability to penetrate the barrier between the brain and blood. This ability makes it possible for much-needed oxygen to be delivered to the brain and stimulate the brain's limbic area – including the hypothalamus, pituitary, and pineal glands. Frankincense produces a warm, thick, creamy, sweet, and balsamic aroma.

In a study done in 2008, it was discovered that one of frankincense essential oil's constituents, incensole acetate, possesses many beneficial qualities including the ability to reduce depressive behavior and anxiety. It is therefore not surprising to find out that the oil has been used for meditation and prayer since ancient times. An extremely versatile oil, frankincense can combine well with practically all types of essential oil.

## 20. Geranium

Pelargonium graveolens is the scientific name of geranium. The essential oil extracted from geranium is known for its potency in relieving stress and tension. Classified as an equalizer and enhancer, it is also known to help release negative memories as it works in tandem with the liver chakra in getting rid of toxins from the body. Geranium oil likewise helps open the mind to accepting new ideas. To gain excellent benefits from the essential oil, it can be diffused or topically applied.

Another versatile essential oil, geranium can be used in combination with any other necessary oil. It exudes a sweet, citrus-rosy, green, and fresh scent. It is recommended that some precautions be observed when using the oil as repeated, and prolonged use can result in some contact sensitization.

## 21. Hyssop

If you study the herb's history, you will learn that hyssop had been regarded as a type of sacred plant that was primarily used as a strewing herb as well as incense to purify sacred or holy places. The essential oil's scent is quite similar to the herb from which it is extracted – sweet, woody, spicy, and healthy.

Hyssop oil, when used in aromatherapy, produces soul-purifying and spirit-refreshing benefits. It combines well with other types of essential oil such as lavender, clove, myrtle, rosemary, clary sage, and sage, as well as citrus oils.

## 22. Jasmine

Jasmine essential oil exudes an intoxicating aroma that uplifts the spirit and promotes the feelings of optimism and confidence. It is, therefore, a great essential oil for relieving depression. Also, it is also recommended to be used when trying to achieve relaxation as well as for insomnia and headache relief. Its scientific name is Jasminum officinale.

Classified as an enhancing, equalizing, and modifying type of essential oil, it can blend well with frankincense, bergamot, lemongrass, Helichrysum, Melissa, mandarin, orange, rose, palmarosa, rosewood, rose, spearmint, and sandalwood. Its scent can be described as sweet, robust, floral, and tenacious. Pure jasmine oil can be very expensive, so you have to make sure that when buying, you get the genuine product and not the synthetic versions that are much cheaper, but a lot less potent.

## 23. Juniper Berry

Juniper berry essential oil is extracted from dried ripe fruits of the juniper tree. It exudes a warm, balsamic, woody pine needle, and fresh aroma. In various consumer products such as outdoorsy and masculine perfumes, spicy colognes, after shaves, and room sprays, juniper berry essential oil is listed as one of the ingredients.

Inhaling juniper through an essential oil diffuser can result in anxiety and stress relief because of its restoring and supportive benefits.

## 24. Lavandin

A hybrid, lavender plant is the product of a natural cross-pollination process between spike lavender and bright purple. Lavandin essential oil possesses a spicy-green camphor-like and woody scent. It is a favorite ingredient in colognes that offer an herbaceous aroma. Lavandin combines well with many types of essential oils including geranium, cypress, cinnamon, clove, citronella, pine, leaf, patchouli, and thyme, among others.

The aroma is not too strong, and it requires a fixative to be added when you need the essential oil to last for several hours. In aromatherapy, lavendin oil produces purifying, balancing, and clarifying effects. Thus, it is ideal to reduce the levels of stress and anxiety.

## 25. Lavender

Arguably the most popular essential oil around, lavender (scientific name Lavendula augustifolia) is considered as the ultimate among adaptogen essential oils. Adaptogens have the capability to balance any personality. In a study conducted in 1988, the ECG patterns of participants who were made to inhale lavender oil were measured. The study subjects said they felt relaxed, and their ECG patterns indicated that they were experiencing certain levels of drowsiness. The participants, however, were able to perform mathematical computations successfully. In fact, they did so in a more accurate and faster fashion.

Simply put, for anxiety and stress relief, lavender essential oil can make you more alert – naturally. Not too many sedatives available in the market can boast of the same benefits. Lavender is classified as a modifier, equalizer, and enhancer. It has a balsamic, sweet, herbaceous, floral scent with hints of woody undertones. It likewise combines well with citrus oils and many other types of essential oils like clary sage, chamomile, and geranium.

## 26. Lemon Balm

The essential oil derived from lemon balm is much more popularly used in Europe for its ability to relieve anxiety and stress than it is in the US. The use of lemon balm as a medicinal herb can be traced to as far back as the Middle Ages.

In a study conducted by a France-based plant extract company, Berkem, the results indicated that anxiety-related symptoms were reduced by as much as 72% after the participants were made to use lemon balm essential oil for an average of 15 days. Similar studies conducted later yielded almost the same results. Lemon balm has likewise been proven to possess antiseptic properties. When using lemon balm, it is best to mix the essential oil with vegetable oil before rubbing into your hands, and then inhaling the aroma.

## 27. Lime

The scientific name for lime is Citrus aurantifolia. The essential oil from lime offers stimulating and invigorating effects that help provide almost instant relief from depression, anxiety, and fatigue.

Lime essential oil combines very well with lavender, clary sage, ylang-ylang, and neroli essential oils. It is best used when experiencing extremely stressful situations and inhaled using an essential oil diffuser.

## 28. Magnolia

The essential oil of Magnolia has properties that help provide relief from anxiety and nervousness. It has a sweet, floral scent. It soothes the mind, eliminates the stress of daily living, and promotes optimism for the future.

Magnolia essential oil is known to combine well with sandalwood, rose, clary sage, and geranium. It is recommended to be used with an essential oil diffuser to achieve optimum benefits for stress and anxiety relief.

## 29. Marjoram

The scientific name of marjoram is Origanum marjorana. The essential oil is classified as an active mood equalizer and enhancer during stressful and anxiety-filled situations. According to folklore marjoram is considered by the Romans as the "happiness herb." The Greeks, on the other hand, referred to the herb as the "pride and joy of the mountains." Aside from its sleep-promoting properties, marjoram essential oil is known for its muscle relaxant, anti-inflammatory, and antispasmodic qualities.

A versatile type of essential oil, marjoram can blend well with cedar wood, bergamot, lavender, cypress, orange, lemongrass, rosemary, nutmeg, ylang-ylang, and rosewood. It possesses a green, herbaceous, and spicy scent. The use of marjoram should be avoided during the entire period of pregnancy.

## 30. Myrrh

The essential oil of myrrh is known to stimulate thoughts and nervous activity, among other health benefits. By stimulating the nervous system and the brain, it keeps the body active and alert. Myrrh is also highly regarded in aromatherapy because of its antidepressant and sedative properties. It is likewise known to enhance feelings of spirituality. Myrrh is also typically recommended for use in relieving symptoms associated with menstruation such as hormonal imbalance and mood swings.

For optimum results, myrrh can be combined with different types of other essential oils like lavender, frankincense, patchouli, palmarosa, sandalwood, rosewood, thyme, and tea tree, among others.

## 31. Myrtle

Myrtle essential oil is extracted from an evergreen shrub that can be found growing wildly all over the Mediterranean. It possesses a uniquely camphor-like and spicy aroma. Experts say that the sweeter the scent of oil, the fresher note it exudes. Myrtle is a favorite ingredient in colognes that offer natural and outdoors-type scents.

Known for its cleansing and clarifying benefits in aromatherapy that soothes anxiety and stress, myrtle blends nicely with other essential oils like lavender, bergamot, clary sage, rosemary, and lime.

## 32. Neroli

Extracted from the orange plant's flower, orange blossom or neroli essential oil is popular for it's relaxing and calming aroma that promotes, sensuality, peace, hopefulness, and confidence. It is known by its scientific name Citrus aurantium bigardia. Orange blossom essential oil may be used with a diffuser or topically applied as a perfume to enjoy its stress-relieving and anxiety-soothing benefits.

Classified as an equalizer, personified, and modifier, Neroli combines well with sandalwood, lavender, rose, cedar wood, jasmine, lemon, and geranium. It possesses a scent that can best be described as sweet, floral, citrusy, slightly bitter, and delicate.

## 33. Nutmeg

Extracted and distilled from dried whole nutmegs, nutmeg essential oil is characterized by the volatile, oily-spicy, and aromatic scent of whole nutmegs. To get the oil, nutmegs are cut into smaller pieces and pressed to get rid of the fixed oil that is more commonly known as nutmeg butter.

Nutmeg essential oil is popularly used as an ingredient in spicy perfumes and men's fragrances. When used in aromatherapy, nutmeg offers relief from anxiety and stress as it uplifts, energizes and rejuvenates a sagging spirit and body.

## 34. Orange

The scientific name of orange essential oil is Citrus sinensis. In a research done in Japan's Mei University, on patients who were treated with orange fragrance, it was shown that the subjects were able to reduce the amount of antidepressant medications they were taking significantly. Likewise, orange essential oil helped restore their immune and endocrine systems back to normal levels. The oil can be taken internally or used with an essential oil diffuser.

Classified as a personified and enhancer, orange blends well with other essential oils like frankincense, juniper, cinnamon bark, geranium, nutmeg, rosewood, and lavender. Its aroma is described as citrusy, fresh, sweet, and fruity. A word of caution, though; when used as a topical application on exposed skin, exposure to direct sunlight must be avoided for no less than 12 hours after application.

## 35. Patchouli

The essential oil of patchouli helps combat anxiety and depression as it balances the emotions and provides relief from lethargy. It likewise helps to enhance imagination and intuition. It can be diluted in vegetable oil for a relaxing massage, added to essential oil diffusers to deodorize a room. Adding 10 - 12 drops of patchouli oil to bath water will help achieve a relaxing bath.

When used in small amounts, the oil can act as a stimulant that provides a quick energy boost, optimism, and vitality. On the other hand, when used in large quantities, it can serve as a sedative that helps calm the nervous system.

## 36. Peru Balsam

Derived from the wild trees that freely grow along El Salvador's "Balsam Coast," Peru balsam emits a delicious, sweet, vanilla-like, and balsamic scent. Considered among the best fixatives around, it has excellent staying power.

When used in aromatherapy, it provides strengthening and anchoring effects that help calm anxious nerves and relieves tension. Peru balsam essential oil combines well with scents that are Oriental, floral, balsamic, and spicy in nature.

## 37. Pine

Pine essential oil is derived from the needles and twigs of the Scotch pine found in abundance in most parts of the Asian and European continents. The aroma is fresh and resinous, unmistakably coming from the pine needle. Pine oil is used to provide a pleasant scent to various personal care and household products like detergents, room sprays, cough and cold preparations, vaporizer liquids, and perfumes for men.

When using the essential oil, make sure that it is diluted well because it can result to skin irritations, especially on sensitive skin. For anxiety and stress relief, it is best used with an essential oil diffuser to achieve refreshing and invigorating effects.

## 38. Rose

Going by the scientific name of Rosa damascena, the rose is one of the most popular essential oils around. It's intense, warm, rosy, and immensely rich scent is associated with love. When used in perfumes, it adds a touch of depth and beauty. It is also a favorite ingredient in powders, lotions, and skin creams. With one or two drops of rose essential oil, you can enjoy a soothing and luxurious bath oil, massage or facial. In aromatherapy, the rose is known to provide supportive, gently uplifting, and romantic effects. It is classified as a personifying, equalizing, modifying, and enhancing essential oil.

Known as a mind stimulant, rose promotes a sense of overall wellbeing. Among all essential oils in its class, it is considered as the one with the highest frequency at 320 MHz. The fragrance of therapeutic grade and pure rose essential oil can be quite overpowering; thus, it is recommended that when using it topically on its own, it should not exceed a slight dab. In general, rose essential oil is best used in combination with other oils, instead of on its own. It blends well with cedar wood cypress, clary sage, frankincense, myrrh, juniper, citrus oils, pine, patchouli, sandalwood, and rosewood. The scent is sensual, dark, rich, spicy, floral, honey-like, and green. Likewise, it should be used with extreme care during pregnancy. As the oil can be very expensive, you must make sure to buy the natural oil and not any of its cheap imitations.

## 39. Rosemary

Rosemary essential oil is commonly called the herb of remembrance. The rosemary plant produces a type of essential oil that can be described as almost colorless but possesses a fresh, camphor-like, and strong scent. It has clarifying and invigorating benefits for anxiety and stress.

The essential oil is a favorite ingredient in Oriental and forest perfumes, as well as in various citrus colognes and eau de cologne. Likewise, dark hair rinses, disinfectants, room deodorants, household sprays, and soaps often list rosemary essential oil as an ingredient.

## 40. Rosewood

Also known as Bois de rose, rosewood is a wild-growing tropical tree found in abundance in the Amazon basin. Its floral-nutmeg and the sweet-woody scent make it a popular ingredient in fantasy-type colognes and perfumes. Likewise, the essential oil is extensively used in scent lotions, soaps, creams, massage and bath oils.

With its calming and gently strengthening benefits, it can help reduce the tension from a stress-filled day. Rosewood is ideally used with an essential oil diffuser.

## 41. Sandalwood

In many cultures around the world, sandalwood (scientific name Santalum album) is used as a meditation and yoga aid. In India, sandalwood essential oil is regarded sacred. It is known to have beneficial effects on the limbic systems of the brain, and it is useful in balancing both the immune system and the emotions.

Classified as an equalizer and modifier, sandalwood essential oil may be topically applied or used with a diffuser. It blends well with other essential oils like spruce, frankincense, cypress, ylang-ylang, myrrh, lemon, and patchouli. Sandalwood produces a scent that can be described as slightly fruity and minty. It should be used with extreme caution during the entire period of pregnancy.

Just like jasmine and rose essential oils, real sandalwood is very expensive because of its currently diminishing supply. Thus, the essential oil is commonly being adulterated and diluted.

## 42. Spikenard

Also known as Nardostachys jatamansi, Spikenard essential oil is rare. It emits an aromatic fragrant oil with hints of musk. It is known in aromatherapy for its ability to promote a Zen-like state and establish inner peace and emotional stability. It is considered as a precious ingredient for various types of massage oils that are used to relieve insomnia, anxiety, and headache. It is also known to release stress from daily living.

Spikenard oil can be combined with other essential oils, specifically lemon, lavender, neroli, clary sage, vetiver, and patchouli.

## 43. Spruce

Spruce essential oil is produced using some evergreen conifer species. It exudes a pleasant, sweet, balsamic, and pine aroma. It is popularly used as an ingredient to lend a fresh pine scent to various household products on its own or in combination with other types of pine needle oils. These products include room sprays, air fresheners, detergents, disinfectants, and soaps.

Spruce essential oil blends well with galbanum, rosemary, and cedar wood, as well as other pine needle essential oils. It offers vitalizing and clarifying effects when used in aromatherapy.

## 44. Tea Tree

The indigenous natives of Australia had long been using tea tree leaves for their many health benefits even long before it was supposedly "discovered" by the men of James Cook, a famous English Explorer. Tea tree essential oil exudes a spicy, warm, subtle, and medicinal aroma; and it is sometimes used to lend fragrance to spicy colognes and aftershave products.

Tea tree oil combines well with other essential oils like rosemary, nutmeg, and lavender. In aromatherapy, the essential oil is known to provide purifying, cleansing, and uplifting effects.

## 45. Thyme

Both the red and white varieties of thyme essential oil are produced from thyme plants that grow in the wild, and are commonly used to scent colognes, aftershaves, and soaps. Thyme essential oil, however, can irritate sensitive skin, and must, therefore, be used with proper caution. In aromatherapy, red and white thyme provides stress relief because of their purifying, cleansing, and energizing properties.

Red Thyme offers a spicy-medicinal, sweet, and herbal aroma, while the white variety exudes a milder aroma and action. White thyme essential oil comes from red thyme oil that has been refined and redistilled further to remove the constituent substances that are responsible for the red color.

## 46. Valerian Root

Valerian root (scientific name Valeriana officialis) Essential oil is famous for the positive effects it has on sleep enhancement. Although not commonly known, the essential oil can likewise be used as a stimulant. Valerian has a scent that may be considered as a bit unpleasant, but it's incredible anxiety-reducing properties cannot be overlooked.

German researchers conducted a study a few years ago on two groups of subjects – one group given benzodiazepine sedatives, and another group administered with valerian essential oil. Both groups showed similar improvements, but the group that was given valerian oil showed significantly fewer unwanted side effects. Valerian root essential oil may be taken orally as a supplement or applied topically on the wrists or soles of the feet. When taken internally, the essential oil must be diluted (1 drop of valerian w/one tsp. of honey, or 4 oz./120 ml of beverage.) It is not recommended for children below six years old.

# 47. Vanilla

According to aromatherapists, the reason why the aroma of warm vanilla makes people feel "right at home" is because, regarding flavor and fragrance, vanilla is the closest that one can get to mothers' milk. No wonder everybody loves vanilla.

Vanilla essential oil's rich aroma has wide-ranging therapeutic effects – from stimulating mental clarity to providing smooth and soothing relaxation. It also provides other health benefits like reducing sweet cravings and relieving an upset stomach.

# 48. Vetiver

The essential oil distilled from vetiver can be described as a very emotionally calming and grounding oil. It can also provide support if you are trying to recover from a recent trauma. Its scent is likewise quite earthy, reminiscent of the woods where watching leaves drop to the ground during fall can be very relaxing.

Vetiver is among the essential oils that have the highest concentrations of sesquiterpenes. In a study conducted by Dr. Terry Friedmann, vetiver essential oil was found to provide significant help in improving behavior in children.

## 49. Wintergreen

In the past, wintergreen essential oil was considered as a crucial material in perfumery and flavoring. However, because of its prohibitive cost, a lot of cheaper and more reliable supplies made from synthetic methyl salicylate have taken its revered place.

While Wintergreen may have lost its popularity among manufacturers of consumer products like mouthwash and toothpaste, it remains a potent aid for stress and anxiety. When used in aromatherapy, it provides bracing, refreshing and invigorating effects.

## 50. Ylang ylang

Ylang ylang (scientific name Cananga oudurata) is known for its potent aphrodisiac qualities and is particularly beneficial for managing anger and stress. Other health benefits that can be enjoyed from inhaling the essential oil's aroma include stimulation of blood circulation and reducing blood pressure. Ylang ylang may be topically applied on the wrists, feet, neck, and back area. It may also be used with a diffuser. The essential oil produces a sweet, cloying, thick, and tropical floral scent with hints of spicy balsamic undertones.

Ylang ylang essential oil has a blend classification of modifier and personified. It is best combined with other oils such as bergamot, anise, chamomile, cardamom, geranium, cumin, lemon, grapefruit, vetiver, sandalwood, and marjoram, instead of being used on its own. If used repeatedly, ylang-ylang oil may result in contact sensitization; hence it must be applied with caution.

# Chapter9:
# ESSENTIALS OILS FOR DETOX AND CLEANING

## Best Essential Oils for Cleaning

### Lemon Essential Oil

Scent: Clean, Fresh, Bright, the staple of any essential oil cleaning kit, starts with lemon essential oils. Naturally antibacterial, lemon is a powerhouse for cutting grease and tackling tough jobs. It's hard to resist the refreshing lemon scent that makes it ideal for air freshening and deodorizing too.

### Orange Essential Oil

Scent: Clean, Sweet, Crisp Harness the strength and aromas of orange essential oils. From your stove, oven, microwave, and everything in between, orange essential oils will tackle the job and have it smelling zesty in no time.

## Tea Tree Essential Oil

Scent: Earthy, Herbal, Woody was also known as Melaleuca, this is the #1 germ fighter when you need to wipe out mold, mildew, and other unmentionables lurking around the house. Tea tree delivers exceptional cleaning results without the laundry list of harmful side effects associated with bleach. Harmful germs and bacteria don't stand a chance when you tackle them with tea tree essential oil.

## Lavender

Lavender tops the list for versatility. It has cleansing and healing properties, and it has been clinically tested for its relaxing properties; both physical and mental.

Lavender also stands above many other essential oils because of its kindness to your skin. It helps to repair skin and keep it elastic and is perfect in homemade anti-aging creams. It is shown to prevent tissue degeneration. It is soothing, and it enhances new cell growth

Lavender also works well when blended with coconut oil to treat rashes like eczema. It is also excellent for treating burns. It promotes healing, reduces pain and minimizes scarring.

We offer several recipes using lavender for bath and skin care. You can also put a few drops in your diffuser to help you unwind and sleep soundly.

Lavender can help you if you suffer from seasonal allergies. Try our Seasonal Allergies Essential Oil Diffuser Recipe.

Lavender also works well if you have dandruff or dry scalp. Just massage a few drops into your scalp. Add lavender to a cotton pad when you store your winter sweaters. It repels moths and eliminates stinky mothballs.

Lavender's lovely aroma also makes it a welcome addition to your laundry regime. Try our Homemade Laundry Detergent.

## Eucalyptus Essential Oil Scent:

Airy, Herbal, and Earthy. Do you want to invigorate your home with a "spa-like" scent? Fresh, clean, and spacious eucalyptus essential oils will bring the feeling of peace and relaxation while it's doing the dirty work for you. Get rid of mold, mildew, and other nasty germs and bacteria with eucalyptus essential oil. Pair with lavender essential oils in laundry and air freshening for an invigorating scent.

**Lemongrass Essential Oil Scent:**

Crisp, Clean, Zesty Lemongrass essential oil is complimented by a refreshing and uplifting scent, along with antibacterial properties. Mix up a lemongrass multi-purpose cleaner, add to your dishwashing detergent, freshen up laundry, and deodorize the whole house. Lemongrass is the perfect

# Essential oil for those that love a spring clean feeling!

Let's get rid of the stockpile of harmful chemical cleaners and make room for your new essential oil filters. This is the first step in making the switch to cleaning with essential oils! It is important to take responsibility to safely remove and dispose of these filters to minimize the adverse effects to yourself and the environment. Improper disposal could lead to contamination producing toxic fumes, chemicals leaching into the groundwater, or destruction of pipelines infrastructure.

# CONCLUSION

This book had introduced you to the world of essential oils, right from the beginnings, when people were merely experimenting with a range of products. It has established a scientific basis for using these products, as well as the inherent challenges of finding the right balance. Ultimately, this book has laid the foundation for any future efforts to professionalize the art and science of aromatherapy. This is an age when we are reconsidering virtually everything that relates to traditional medicine. It is, therefore, not surprising that remedies, which were once dismissed as being nothing more than amateurish science, have come to dominate the market. In fact, essential oils have led to the development of new professions that were previously considered to be unworkable. Moreover, these oils allow people to treat their conditions in a way that is safe, cost-effective, and efficient. The book readily acknowledges the fact that it is not always easy to get the best out of the products marketed as essential oils. For example, there are many potential side effects, depending on the health of the person and the way they use the product. Moreover, the fact that there is very limited information about the potential benefits and downsides of these oils means many people are, effectively, operating in darkness. To bring balance to the book, there is no claim that essential oils are the solution to all the ailments of humanity. Rather, the argument is that this is an alternative solution for people, who want to think outside the box.

The next stage is to start thinking about how you can apply these essential oils in your life. The first part is to read books, such as this one, so you are well versed in the subject and its implications. Then, you can start with a few conventional oils in very dilute forms to test how your body reacts to them. With confidence, you can expand your horizons by using more complex oils and blends. This book will be a major reference point throughout the process. The book is, by no means, exhaustive, and you may have to supplement a lot of the information it contains. Nevertheless, this book has broadly achieved the objectives with which it started. Here, you have an overview of the origins and basics of essential oils, so readers can be inspired to explore the topic further. As for the prospects for the industry, they seem excellent. Many more people are overcoming their traditional prejudices against alternative medicine. They increasingly see it as a way of countering some of the worst impacts of the conventional methods. In practice, that experimental beginning has not meant it to be a free fall. Indeed, many governments set out stringent criteria for what is and what is not an essential oil. These rules are there for your safety, as a consumer. That is why this book has emphasized the need for care and precaution when using essential oils. Nevertheless, this is a fun way to develop healthful living habits. If you get it right, then you could be able to get rid of some ailments that are not responding to conventional medicine. Try the essential oils today and see what they can do for you.

You now know about many of the different types of essential oils that are available to you, as well as some of the most commonly used carrier oils. After reading through this book, you are aware of many of the uses that essential oils have, as well as how to utilize the oils to accomplish many different health and beauty results.

You have also learned about all of the other applications essential oils can have in your life. Remember that many of the things that require the use essential oils only require a few drops, which makes it easy to replace many of the products in your home with essential oils, and save yourself a lot of time and money.

The next thing for you to do is decide which recipe you want to try first. Remember you aren't limited to the methods that we have provided here for you. With the information, you now have on carriers and essential oils, you have the information you need to make whatever you want with your essential oils!

Thank you for purchasing this book I hope you will apply the acquired knowledge productively.